Mental Illness of Incarcerated Population

Mental Illness of Incarcerated Population

Ruby Sisk, M.A.

Copyright © 2018 by Ruby Sisk, M.A..

ISBN:	Softcover	978-1-9845-3234-3
	eBook	978-1-9845-3233-6

All rights reserved. No part of this book may be reproduced or transmitted in any form or by any means, electronic or mechanical, including photocopying, recording, or by any information storage and retrieval system, without permission in writing from the copyright owner.

The information, ideas, and suggestions in this book are not intended as a substitute for professional medical advice. Before following any suggestions contained in this book, you should consult your personal physician. Neither the author nor the publisher shall be liable or responsible for any loss or damage allegedly arising as a consequence of your use or application of any information or suggestions in this book.

Any people depicted in stock imagery provided by Getty Images are models, and such images are being used for illustrative purposes only.
Certain stock imagery © Getty Images.

Print information available on the last page.

Rev. date: 06/05/2018

To order additional copies of this book, contact:
Xlibris
1-888-795-4274
www.Xlibris.com
Orders@Xlibris.com
780323

Contents

Mental Illness 1
Screening 9
Treatment and Services 17
Reentry of Mentally Ill Inmates 25
Promoting Proactive Partnerships 37

Endnotes 43

Mental Illness

A mental illness is defined as having a psychiatric condition, usually characterized by an impairment of an individual's normal cognitive, emotional, or behavioral functioning. This is caused by physiological or psychosocial factors. Also known as mental disease A health condition that changes a person's thinking, feelings, or behavior (or all three) and that causes the person distress and difficulty.

A number of inmates display the classic signs and symptoms of Post Traumatic Stress Disorder (PTSD). An individual with PTSD has been exposed to a traumatic event in which both of the following have been present: The person has experienced, witnessed, or been confronted with an event or events that involve actual or threatened death or serious injury, or threat to the physical integrity of oneself or others. Second, the person's response involved intense fear, helplessness, or horror (Whitefield, 2004).

Overcrowding increases the violence and makes life inside miserable for everyone, especially for prisoners with traumatic pasts who are suffering from PTSD and other serious mental illnesses. A large number of prisoners come from low income, high crime neighborhoods, and have experienced repeated and prolong trauma since childhood. Men who witnessed violence between their parents are three times more likely to commit domestic violence than those who grew up in less abusive homes (Kupers, 1999).

Not all inmates who grow up in high crime neighborhoods develop symptoms of PTSD but a large number avoid psychiatric disability and the criminal justice system altogether, it remains the case that a disproportionate number get into serious trouble. (Kupers, 1999)

PTSD has presented itself in many guises throughout history. In the late 1800's and early 1900's, during the time of Janet, Freud and their colleagues, the term was called hysteria and was seen most often with traumatized young women. During World Wars I and II, it was seen most often in young men and was called shell shock or combat neurosis. Even though children have been physically and otherwise abused for years it was recognized in 1962 as the battered child syndrome. This was considered a guise as well. Another guise was recognized in 1983 as the dysfunctional families, occurring often in people with mental and physical disorders (Whitefield, 2004).

Concern regarding reentry

With the growth of prison population since 1980, prison crowding in most state and federal facilities is getting worse. Many prisons are filled to 150 or 200% of their design capacity (Kupers, 1999). The crowding in prisons increases the violence, psychiatric disturbances and suicide. People, who are prone to impulsive behavior, rule-breaking, and psychiatric disturbances, do not perform well in crowded places. The rise in violence creates many new traumas, especially for the vulnerable, mentally disordered inmates.

Prisoners with mental disorders are segregated when they misbehave. They are punished with time in the "hole." This area is where the mental illness has an opportunity to rise and inmates are at that point manic, meaning they are experiencing the symptoms of the mental illness such as Schizophrenia (Kupers, 1999). Thinking abstractly, feeling worthless, and passiveness with withdrawal and hallucinations are part of the behavior. During this time, there is no treatment for the inmate.

The sanitation and hygiene as well as other harsh conditions of prisons also affect an inmate. Such conditions as flushed waste backing up into the cell neighbor's toilet, no hot water for showering, unclean kitchen for food services, and roaches, in addition, trigger the mental illness symptoms of inmates on the inside. This has increased the inmates' chances of having a heightened reoccurring episode.

In Ruiz v. Estelle[1], a 1980 class action lawsuit, Texas prisoners sued the state for violating their constitutional rights by confining them in excessively harsh conditions and depriving them of adequate mental health care. The federal district court formulated six components of a minimally adequate mental health treatment program:

1. A systematic screening procedure
2. Treatment that entails more than segregation and supervision
3. Treatment that involves a sufficient number of mental health professionals to adequately provide

services to all prisoners suffering from serious mental disorders

4. Maintenance of adequate and confidential clinical records
5. A program for identifying and treating suicidal inmates
6. A ban on prescribing potentially dangerous medications without adequate monitoring (Kupers, 1999).

The quality of care ordered by the courts and mandated standards are designed to "the standard of care in the community" (Kupers, p.68). The inmates are lacking the proper and efficient mental health care treatment and services on the inside. The minimum quality is not enough to fulfill the mental health services to even remotely compare to what is offered upon reentry.

This problem is common upon re-entry into the community, because there is lack of treatment services for the mental ill inmate on the outside. The problems associated with lack of medical care insurance, not being on any type of assistance like Title 19, Social Security, Workman compensation or something that will cover the expenses of their treatment services. The community's feeling on re-entry is that the individuals who are considered for discharge into the community should not be entitled to the same benefits as un-incarcerated persons, because the community feels the inmates have not paid their way to earn this benefit in society (American Association for Correctional Psychology, 2002).

The lack of resources to re-entry is limited and scarce. This is due to the lack of attention the criminal justice and social services systems have involved their agencies with the process to work together to make it a working dual system. The re-entry population needs both agencies to properly guide them through the walk of connections, mainly with the needs of mental health and readjustment into the community mainstreams.

Individuals with psychiatric disabilities are identified and referred to community organizations and mental health and case management services for assessment, evaluation, monitoring and intervention, but the linkages are usually on a voluntary basis. Although mental health counseling may help ex-inmates cope with their re-adjustment to community living and all the expectations, not all ex-inmates with mental illness will have access or will participate in counseling and treatment. (Healey, 1999).

Having benefits in place at the time of release can balance the needs of ex-inmates in the community, by ensuring funds for health and living. For example, Social Security can create the difference between homelessness and being housed. Medicaid can assist with prescriptions. (Jencks, 1994). This helps with the transition of reentry because it helps to overcome some of the barriers.

In essence the need for effective and efficient reentry programs will help to assist individuals with their transition into the community as well as assisting them with the resources for mental health benefits. This will aid the re-occurrences of offending and prevent the cycle of mental episodes, particularly the outbursts that cause mental deviant behavior.

Screening

Early detection of mental disorders is a crucial part of any mental health treatment program because the longer a severe disorder is left untreated, the more severe the symptoms (Kupers, 1999). Screening is a method for identifying arrestees who require emergency attention in prison; however, an assessment is to carry out to determine whether there is a medical or psychiatric condition that warrants attention. The assessment is performed at the reception center within the prison; this is where new prisoners are sent until they can be classified in regard to security level and assigned to a specific institution and cellblock.

Most local jails provide psychiatric screening when detainees are admitted and provisions are made to treat offenders who are ill or at risk. Mental health staffs are assigned to treat prisoners who are found to be suicidal or suffer from mental disorders. Screening procedures are effective only if carried out in a consistent manner (Kupers, 1999).

The American Medical Association and many state governments began to publish standards for the provision of health and mental health services in local detention facilities, including the requirement that screening occur at the time of admission to jail. The screening should include questions designed to rule out the possibility the arrestee is suffering from a critical medical condition or is prone to suicide. (Kupers, 1999).

Screening procedures can provide information about the inmates history for instance if the inmate has a history of mental illness and other health problems that the staff should be concerned with. Staff should obtain assessment and treatment history information from community mental health treatment providers. The individual in charge of conducting the screening is often the booking or receiving officer, intake nurse, or intake clinician; in general, any properly trained individual can administer a screening. The staff should always respect the protocol for obtaining the information. The Criminal Justice/Mental Health

Consensus Project 127 recommended the procedure. The intake personnel, upon receiving an inmate, should perform fingerprinting and do a medical exam in addition to reviewing a host of issues in order to make decisions about classification, programs and special accommodations (Criminal justice/Mental Health Consensus Project, 2009).

There are four levels of services provided upon admissions. The first is referral. This process is utilized for those inmates who appear to be in need of mental health treatment. They receive targeted assessment or evaluation so they can be assigned to appropriate services. Intake screening is second and a comprehensive examination that is performed on each new arrival within fourteen days of arrival. This includes a review of the medical screening, behavior observation, and inquiry into any mental health history, and an assessment of suicide potential.

The third level of the process is the Comprehensive mental health evaluation. This is a face- to- face interview of the person and a review of all reasonably available health care record collateral information. Fourth, if a treatment plan is all ready in existence then the initial treatment plan is re modified and the decision to add to it is determined at the assessment intake level. (American Association for Correctional Psychology).

In prison it is not easy to determine an inmate with mental illness that is why state laws require an assessment which helps in the determination of an inmate with mental illness. The following education for correctional staff teaches them how to access mental illness in the inmates by implementing courses like PSY201: "Supervising Offenders with Mental Illness," (Council of State Governments Justice Center, 2002). This program targets the training needs identified in the Consensus Project Report.

The course is designed for correctional officers who work in jails and prisons on the federal, state, and local levels. It is applicable to correctional supervisors and managers who want a basic review of the subject. It provides an understanding of mental illness and describes how the correctional environment influences offenders with mental disorders. The course discusses how to identify and respond to the signs of mental illness, supervise offenders with mental disorders effectively, prevent and respond to suicides and crises, and participate in the treatment process.

The New York State Office of Mental Health (OMH) and other state departments have partnered on an evidence –based practice initiative that those officials hope will become a national model. The new pilot program, Wellness Self Management (WSM), is being coordinated by the center for Urban Community Services (CUCS) along with OMH and the New York State Department of Corrections and Department of Parole Services, to provide 126 inmates with mental illness among the three state correctional facilities as well as train 35 OMH and New York State Department of Correctional Services Staff (American Association for Correctional Psychology, 2002).

The program will assist in offering tools that may assist an individual to manage the stress associated with every day events, provide education on the symptoms of their diagnosis, in addition to offering the individual skills to assist him or her with overcoming barriers and pursuing personal goals. Among the strategies used within the prison system, inmates will be taught skills for better management of their mental illness, managing life while incarcerated, and transition to the community, reduction in disciplinary actions while incarcerated and work on site in correctional facilities.

This training will give the inmate education to what could lead to a successful discharge. By gaining the knowledge and awareness of their diagnosis and learning how to better control it, will make the transition easier and faster from prison to reentry into the community. The overall goal to get the staff and the individual the education needed for preparation from day one of admittance to jail throughout the inmates process upon reentry, that is why effective screening is necessary to make determinations about the individuals life after a crime has been committed. Decisions of what is next for that individual should be followed up with programs and services.

The integration of criminal justice and the mental health agencies can provide transition planning and assist jail inmates with co-occurring disorders with mechanisms to create interconnected network services. This will provide management information systems with information sharing as permitted by confidentiality requirements and staff training. Working partnerships with probation, neighborhood business and services providers can also develop opportunities for the released offender to participate in restorative and therapeutic activities and community service projects (Austin, J., & Lawson, R., 1998).

The APIC model for jail transition to community is the approach that prioritizes elements for fast track (i.e., less than 72 hours) detainees. The "A" represents assess, meaning assessing the inmate's clinical and social needs, and public safety risks. The "P" represents the plan for treatment and services required to address the inmate's needs. The "I" represents identify required community and correctional programs responsible for post release services. And the "C" represents coordinate the transition plan to ensure implementation and avoid gaps in care with community- based services (Dvoskin, J. &Steadman, H.J. 1994).

Treatment and Services

When inmates with mental illness are no longer under supervision of the criminal justice system they must maintain contact with mental health services and supports for as long as necessary. They must have access to services they need to reintegrate into community settings. The importance of collaboration between mental health and community corrections agencies in ensuring that individuals with mental illness who are granted supervised release receive appropriate mental health services. The policy addresses the role of the mental health system in providing services and support for individuals released from prison who are no longer under supervision from the criminal justice system. This group includes those who have completed their sentence in prison or jail and are released without conditions as well as those who have successfully met the conditions of release and are no longer under supervision in the community (Criminal Justice/Mental Health Consensus Project).

In light of the high recidivism rates of offenders with mental illness, it is crucial that the mental health system maintain contact with individuals who have been incarcerated to prevent their renewed involvement with the criminal justice system. Offenders have basic needs for housing and supports that must be adequately met if reentry is to succeed. Community mental health providers can play an important role in successful community reintegration of former prisoners who have mental illness.

Community mental health providers must be in tuned to the special needs and circumstances of released offenders with mental illness and provide services that enhance their ability to live independently. Developed treatment plans must meet the fit of the offenders and their circumstances (Criminal Justice/Mental Health Consensus Project).

Mental health providers should meet the challenges related to the transition to the community life, such as treatment and rehabilitative models like Assertive

Community Treatment. This transition addresses the problems that could lead to re-arrest (Criminal Justice/ Mental Health Consensus Project, 1997). Special attention should be given from the outset to provision of rehabilitative services that will both address specific needs and help establish a routine for the released offender attempting to grow accustomed to new freedom.

Mental health providers have to be aware of the histories of offenders which differ from non-offenders; additional incentives to engage in care will have to be considered (Criminal Justice Mental Health Consensus Project, 1999).

It is important the programs be developed to meet the specific needs of offenders with mental illness who are transitioning from prison to the community. Correctional settings have had the responsibility for screening and identification of mental health issues as well as for providing treatment while inmates are incarcerated. Opportunities for the released offender to participate in restorative and therapeutic activities and community service projects. The transition planning is important for offenders who will not be under community supervision as it is for those who will have some conditions placed on their release. Programs need to develop a broad selection of services that can be matched to offender needs. The service should include housing, health care, medications, case management, employment, income supports and entitlements. Food and clothing, transportation, and child care (Roskes & Feldman, 1999).

Mental health providers should also consider a support peer group; this will help the offender understand they are not alone. This provides a social network for peers to share their experiences of reentry (Council of State Governments Justice Center, 2002).

Income supports and entitlements, access to mental health and addiction services and the income support that can pay for housing and other services is, for most jail inmates with mental illnesses, available only through public benefits. Medicaid, Social Security/Social Security Disability, veterans, food stamp, and Assistance to Needy Family benefits should be initiated while the person is incarcerated. The courts, probation department, and jail mental health staff should work with local departments of social services, and other agencies that manage health benefits to avoid termination of benefits when an inmate enters jail. Temporary suspension of benefits should occur when the person is admitted to jail. But this rarely happens.

Transitional and aftercare programs help offenders move successfully from more to less restrictive environments in the prison, from prison to parole supervision, and from parole supervision to community reintegration (Rice & Harris, 1993). The goal of reducing the number of parolees with mental health needs, who commit new crimes or violate their parole, depends in part on the availability of aftercare services. The importance of community based mental health care as a condition of parole for offenders.

Current State Programs

Cook County Illinois, in dealing with the Adult Probation Department's Mental Health Unit, has been recognized by the American Probation and Parole Association as the best practice in community corrections. The unit consists of five probation offers and one supervisor, each with a background in mental health. Officers spend the majority of their time monitoring their caseloads, which are smaller than standard probation caseloads. Clients can be referred to the unit by judges or other probation officers working in Chicago and in surrounding suburban court locations (Lurigio & Martin, 1998).

The probation officers refer probationers for mental health services, matching them with treatment facilities and changing services if a different treatment is needed. They assist in the resources and support they need for the alternate treatment program.

California provides specialized services for mentally ill parolees through five Parolee Outpatient Clinics and a Conditional Release Program know as (CONREP). These operate in San Diego, Los Angeles, San Francisco, Sacramento, and Fresno. The clinics serve mentally ill parolees and are staffed by licensed psychiatrists and psychologists.

CONREP is a small successful community based program for offenders who are transferred from prisons to state hospitals and to outpatient psychiatric programs as a condition of parole. Participants must have been in mental health treatment in prison for 90 days or more during the past year and must be assessed as a substantial risk to public safety (Neito, 1999). The parolees are held to conditions of release and receive mental health care in the community.

Baltimore, Maryland developed a specialized mental health program in 1996 for mentally ill offenders on federal probation, parole supervised release, or conditional release in the community. The services consist of psychiatric and medical interventions, drug treatment, assertive case management, urine toxicology screening, and integrated programs for offenders with substance abuse and dependence disorders (Roskes & Feldman, 2000). The program's mental health team routinely exchanges information about clients' progress. Staff coordinates their responses to offenders' failures to treatment or other conditions of release; usually, a therapeutic intervention is a sanction in response to their failure.

For parole services to be successful in the supervision of persons with mental illness, they must address the broad range of offender needs. This does not mean that Parole agencies must provide all of these services. They must, collaborate with the community services agencies that provide mental health and other human services (Veysey, 1996).

In order for the offender to have a successful reentry, services and treatment must be made an intricate part of the person's recovery while in prison and upon the release into the community. The person's reentry should be a healthy transition for adaptation of what the offender is going to face in the community. The training will assist the offenders with social and economic challenges that they need to be prepared for at any given time of their lives, whether they are offenders or not. It is necessary for survival reasons.

Reentry of Mentally Ill Inmates

Reentry describes programs and services designed to help former prisoners successfully reintegrate into communities following their release from jails and prisons and to address the multiple problems that they experiences. Prisoners often experience problems when reentering communities, including substance abuse, mental illness, HIV and AIDS, lack of education, unemployment, homelessness, legal issues to receiving public services such as bans on obtaining public assistance, public housing restrictions and limited transitional housing options, and difficulty obtaining state issued identification (National Governors, Association,

2005). Because of the existing problems of poverty, racism, and community social disorder, many people released from prisons often find themselves caught in environments with too few options for making or sustaining successful reentry.

In the past years, parole agents have had access to relatively scarce resources for offender services and have been responsible for managing large caseloads of releases under conditions of supervision. In a survey of parole agencies, Camp and Camp (1997), for example, found that 64% assisted parolees with job training and development, 32% had drug detoxification services, 59% had drug treatment programs, but none provided specialized mental health services. As a result of caseloads, more stringent conditions of release, and fewer services, an unprecedented number of persons fail on parole and return to prison for violations. Sixty five percent of all of California's prison admissions were parole violators (Austin & Lawson, 1998).

In the Bureau of Justice Statistics annual survey of adult probationers, nearly 548,000 offenders were identified as mentally ill, at the end of 1998 (Ditton, 1999). Probationers as mentally ill reported that they had experienced an "emotional condition" or had been admitted overnight in a mental hospital or mental health facility. A majority of mentally ill probationers were sentenced for public order or property crimes. Compared with none mentally ill probationers, a higher percentage of mentally ill probationers were sentenced for violent crimes, and a lower percentage of them were sentenced for drug crimes.

Parole agents should find alternative strategies for handling the technical violations of releases with mental illnesses. In Veysey's (1996) words, "if community supervision staff adhere to rigid sanctions for technical violations with regard to treatment compliance, special-needs clients particularly those with mental illness are likely to fail" (p. 158). Violations are often a junction of clients' symptoms or their difficulties in following directions. A failure to report, for example, might result from cognitive impairment, delusions, confusion, or side effects of psychotropic medications (Veysey, 1996). As a rule, incarceration or other harsh penalties should be avoided when responding to such instances. More effective options in relapse prevention techniques and systems of progressive sanctions. Parole officers can view technical violations as opportunities to build closer alliances with offenders and assist them in avoiding future and more serious, problems including criminal activity (Nieto, 1999).

This will close the gap and increase the consistency of services provided by way of the assistance of the parole officer.

The National Coalition for Mental and Substance Abuse Health Care in the Justice System stated, "building lasting bridges between the mental health and criminal justice systems, leading to coordinated and continual health care for clients of both systems; involve clients in treatment decisions, ensure public safety as well as the safety of offenders; facilitate the successful integration of offenders into the community; promote offender responsibility and self sufficiency; permit equal access to all health care services, including medical, psychiatric, substance abuse and psychological interventions; avoid discriminating against or stigmatizing mental illness, accommodate clients with multiple needs and problems; be sensitive and responsive to the special needs of mentally ill people of color by developing diverse, culturally sensitive programs; require families to be involved in treatment and supervision plans on mental illness match services and treatments to clients specific problems and needs and raise public awareness about mental illness in the criminal justice system (Lurigio, 1996).

Continuity of Care

This is aftercare planning and liaison work between prison mental health staff and their counterparts in the community. The majority of prisoners, including those with severe and persistent mental disorders, will eventually serve their full sentence and be releases. Some will recycle between community treatment agencies and correctional facilities. As part of the treatment plan inside prison, social workers or other outreach liaison workers must remain in touch with the prisoner's families; work with agencies in the community, and do all that is possible to facilitate a smooth transition to post- release life in the community. A prison treatment program is not really viable if it does not provide comprehensive post release services (Kupers, 1999). The continuity of care will include the entitlements of programs that will serve as the bases for the care and treatment of the mental ill offender population. People with mental illness are admitted to jails and prisoners each year and many of them may be eligible for federal benefits or entitlement programs such as Medicaid, Supplemental Security Income, and Social Security Disability Insurance upon release from jail or prison. Enrollment in the programs can improve access to mental health and other services and supports which, in turn, facilitate compliances with conditions of release. This increases public safety and reduces spending on jails and prisons (Henry, 2004). Many case managers working with correctional facilities lack resources to assist offenders with mental illness in applying for benefits or reinstating. Prison administrators and other officials may be unsure as well as to how to initiate better discharge planning for offenders needing assistance of public benefits. Key policies are recommended along with state background information to aid in the assistance planning.

The focus on Medicaid/SSI/SSDI benefits access offenders with mental illness returning from jail and prison can help with health care, housing and essential supports. The recommendations are to help corrections directors, human services, and social security officials and other representatives overseeing policy decisions that affect offenders with mental illness returning from the criminal justice system review policy recommendations in areas of eligibility, documentation, applications and continuity of care. This will be reviewed and implemented by interagency groups with representatives from corrections departments, state agencies overseeing Medicaid, and mental health and local regional Social Security offices. This tool outlines policies that are relevant to offenders with mental illness in jail or prison who may be eligible for the Medicaid assistance upon release (Henry, 2004).

Impact on the Community

Proclamations were made to assure the public that by keeping more serious offenders behind bars for longer periods of time, criminals would be receiving their "just desserts" or bad guys would stop being let out of prison early, and communities would be safer. This message resonated with citizens and lawmakers. By 1998, 14 states abolished early prison release by parole board authority, and several others restricted the use of parole (Ditton & Wilson, 1999). A number of states also eliminated or curtailed parole supervision but later reinstated discretionary release mechanisms and monitoring services that the length of prison sentence served had actually decreased following the elimination of parole and the ability to provide surveillance or treatment of high risk offenders (Petersilia, 1999). With this information given, it made it possible for offenders of high risk to be released into the community with monitoring. This forced communities to have to live as neighbors with mental ill offenders released into the community.

The Forensic Transition Team, Massachusetts Department of Mental Health established in 1998 designed a transitional release planning services for offenders to release offenders from correctional custody to community. The team consults the community providers for up to three months after release to address any obstacles to client community adjustment arrangements of programs, treatments, and social support services. The criminal justice officials address public safety concerns with institutional corrections authorities and with probation and parole officials to coordinate the linkages for offenders with mental illness to receive community based services upon release. (Criminal Justice Mental Health Consensus Project, 1997). The strategy is to have the transition planner working with the inmate during the last months of their incarceration and facilitating the person's compliance with conditions of release after the offender is released to the community (Council of State Governments Justice Center, 2002). Corrections system has developed different approaches to ensure that an inmate's release into the community is gradual. Some of these programs involve assignment to a pre- release housing unit within a minimum security unit or in a community based setting. Correctional discharge planners assigned to these programs help make community contacts and referrals for housing, employment, and services. Transition planners' responsibilities include assessing offenders' needs and strengths and facilitating appropriate community based services. The special needs of these populations' transition planners need to be aware of what services are available in the jurisdictions they serve and which community and treatment of people with mental illness (Criminal Justice/Mental Health Consensus Project, 1997).

Provisions upon Release

States have a statute or a constitutional amendment requiring the victim be notified before the offender is releases from prison. Regardless of whether the inmate to be released has a mental illness, releasing authorities and correctional staff must comply with victim notification requirements (Criminal Justice Mental Health Consensus Project, 1997). Efforts should be made through correctional crime victim specialists and community based crime victim agencies to reach out to crime victims and inform them of the pending release date of those who have victimized them, to educate them as to the decisions being made on behalf of the offender, and to provide them information about the measures being taken to ensure their safety.

Monitor the inmate closely in the days approaching release and modify the discharge plan when appropriate. Successful implementation of the transition plan is usually on the following: updated examinations on the inmate's mental health and psychotropic medications requirements on the release date, cooperation among at least two agencies to enable representatives from one agency to navigate another system credibly, and provision of a mental health status evaluation for the purpose of risk assessment and supervision. (Kupers, 1999). A mental health professional should conduct a mental health assessment of the inmate at a point just prior to release to ensure that the discharge plan is fully adequate to addressing the inmate's current needs and circumstances. If this is not done, the mental health professional should work with the releasing authority to modify the discharge plan accordingly (Criminal Justice/Mental Health Consensus Project, 1997).

Given the public health and public safety issues associated with reentry, developing policies that promote successful reentry not only are needed, but also are essential for a "healthy" nation. In the current economic environment, one might observe that the criminal justice system is one of the few "growing" sectors. A society that is not doing everything possible to reverse the alarming trends in incarceration and recidivism must not be a society invested in the health and mental health of all of its citizens (Draine, 2005).

Reentry affects communities in disproportionate ways, African American males are incarcerated at seven times the rate of white men, and eight of every ten African American males will be incarcerated at some point during their lives (Lotke, 1998). For many African American males and men of color, the criminal justice system is a harsh reality. This reality is often accompanied with social stressors that compound health and mental health concerns and issues that social workers must address. The benefits of addressing these issues can be found not only at the individual level, but also at the community level and go a long way in dealing with the social disorder that frames the lives of these men (Draine, 2005). The data suggest that some communities are vulnerable to reentry and the problems associated with returning prisoners (Hughes &Wilson, 2002). Reentry affects ethnic minority communities in terms of children and families, inadequate access to health care, housing, and higher education, immigration status, employment, voting rights, and drug use. The issues listed are why people should be concerned about reentry and the importance of proactive partnerships with state and local agencies.

Promoting Proactive Partnerships

In President Bush 2004 State of the Union address he proposed a four year demonstration grant program that allocated $300 million for the Prisoner Reentry Initiative (PRI). The services intended to strengthen urban communities and reduce recidivism were provided by faith based and community organizations that included job training and placement, transitional housing services, mentoring assistance and other transitional services for former prisoners (U.S. Department of Labor, 2007).

During the first year of the program, 30 grantees provided 43,495 services to 6,442 former prisoners, and

3,378 former prisoners obtained employment (U.S. Department of Labor, 2007). Early data describing PRI recidivism rates are promising and show that the recidivism rate was 20% representing less than one- half the Bureau of Justice's statistics national figure of 44% (Faith- based and community initiatives, 2004).

Vocational training and work release programs were effective for reducing recidivism and improving job readiness skills; drug treatment was effective for reducing drug use, recidivism, drug related crimes, and parole violations; educational programs increased educational achievement scores, but did not decrease recidivism; halfway house programs reduced severe criminal behavior; and prerelease programs reduced recidivism (Hartwell, 2005). The need for the coordination of community services organized around the realities facing the reentry population; health, mental health, employment, housing, and substance abuse gives the need for a variety of services.

A critical examination of the roles, functions, and outcomes of U.S. criminal justice programs and policies, they can create a system in which recidivism for many incarcerated people is commonplace, if not f foregone conclusion (Golder et al., 2005) provided a comprehensive examination of factors that support successful reentry with a focus on mental health practice with adults. The work needs social workers and other professionals to develop their knowledge of evidence- based practices. Social workers can use this knowledge in developing programs that sustain individuals in community settings where they are not just released into a waiting place for return to the incarcerated environment (Freudenberg, 2006).

In 2000, the leaders of community organizations in Jefferson County, Colorado, came together with state officials to tackle problems of reentry. The partners were determined to develop a way to provide cost effective community based mental health services for offenders with mental illness who are leaving prison to keep them from reoffending an ending back in the criminal justice system. The collaborating agencies researched programs nationwide to develop a service delivery plan. The result was the John Eachon Reentry Program (JERP). The goal is to decrease recidivism and reduce the length of incarceration by providing community -based therapeutic services and responding to the community transition needs of offenders with serious mental illness.

The program is characterized by a continuity of treatment, access to medication during the transition out of prison and into the community, and collaborative team-based case management, all of which enhance the likelihood that program participants will effectively reenter the community. (Rice & Harris, 1993).

Eachon was an executive manager at the Jefferson Center who died of cancer while JERP was being developed. He is remembered for his leadership in fostering local collaborations to address unmet mental health needs in the community. It was his first dedication and commitment to finding the "common ground" for interagency service providers working to improve the lives of persons with mental illness, as well as his work on the program's development, that inspired the JERP Committee. The Jefferson Center is JERP's lead agency. The Jefferson County and state agencies also provide in kind and financial contributions totaling an estimation of $371, 650 per year. (Hall, 2008).

JERP annually provides 30 to 45 parolees with transitional housing (a halfway house for offenders) or residential treatment. (Hall, 2008). The program offers comprehensive, individual mental health and substance abuse treatment, along with correctional supervision services. A multidisciplinary team consisting of a case manager, parole officer, two mental health professionals, and medical staff members provide assessment, evaluation, and services to offenders.

The first two years of JERP have proven to be highly effective in achieving the objectives of successfully reintegrating consumers into the community and meeting the challenges inherent in working with this population (Hall, 2008).

The Mentally Ill Offender Treatment and Crime Reduction Act of 2004, will improve access to mental health services for adult and juvenile non- violent offenders, was signed into law by the President on October 30. On October 6, the U.S. House of Representatives passed the bill and the Senate followed on October 11. "This law places critical resources where they are needed most, on the front lines," says Russ Newman, Ph. D., J.D., APA's executive director for professional practice. This will improve collaboration among the criminal justice, juvenile justice, and mental health and substance abuse treatment systems. It will ensure that both adult and juvenile non violent offenders with mental health disorders are identified properly and reccive the treatment they need from the point of arrest to reentry into the community, and are not simply recycled into the system. This legislation authorizes a $50 million federal grant program for states and counties to establish more mental health courts, expand prisoners' access to mental health treatment while incarcerated and upon reentry into the community, provide additional resources for pre-trial jail diversion programs and related initiatives, and fund cross-training for law enforcement officials and mental health personnel dealing with adult and juvenile offenders with mental health disorders. The new law, recognizing the needs of offenders with mental health disorders, is consistent with the recommendations of President Bush's New Freedom Commission on Mental Health in 2002 which cited jail diversion and community reentry programs. (American Psychology Association, 2009).

Endnotes

[1] In 1980 a class action suit in Texas, Ruiz v. Estelle, federal decisions established specific criteria for constitutionally adequate psychiatric care in jails and prisons (American Psychiatric Association, 2000).

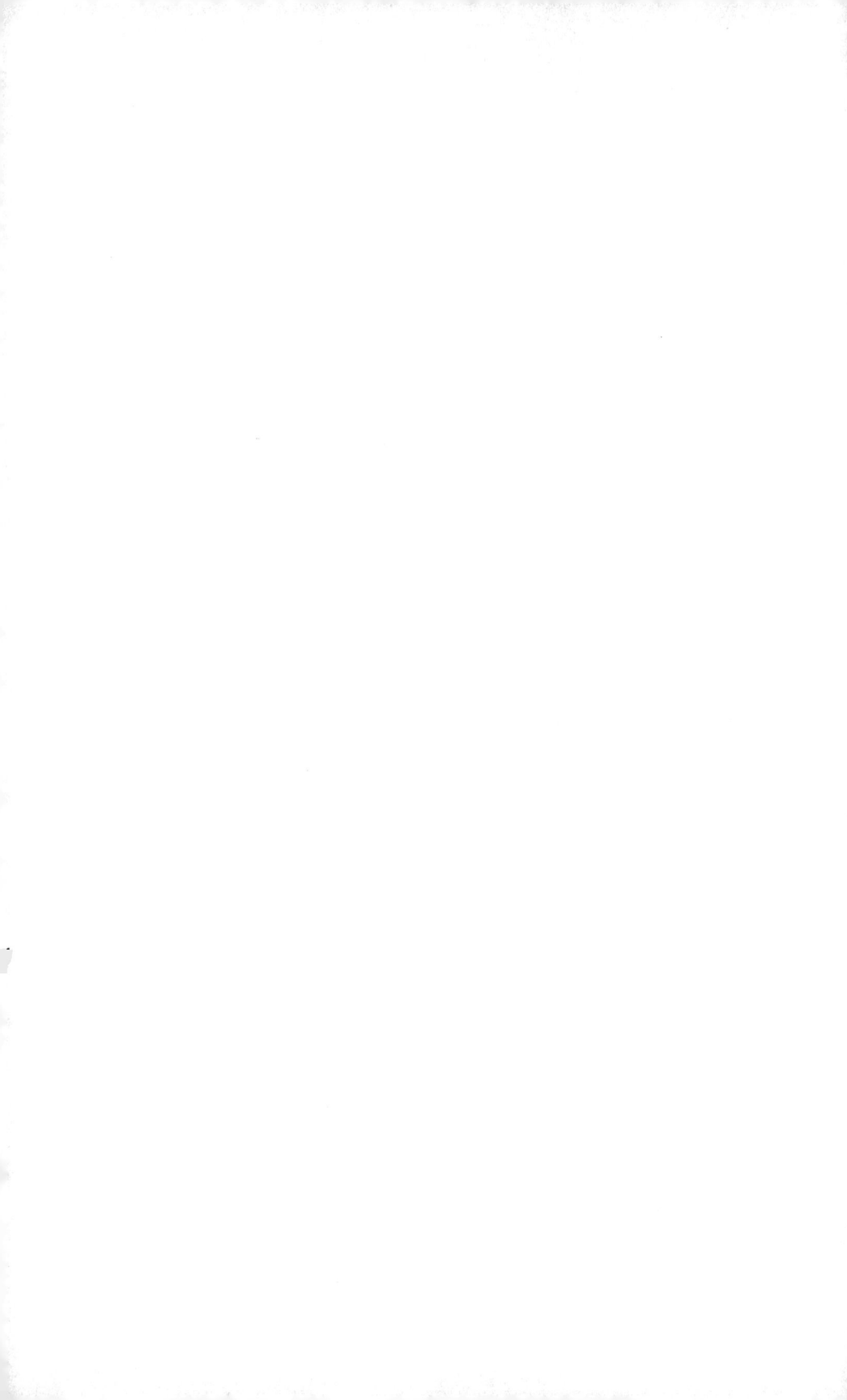

www.ingramcontent.com/pod-product-compliance
Lightning Source LLC
Chambersburg PA
CBHW031553210526
45464CB00003B/1287